REJECT THE DIET MENTALITY

What Kind Of Eater Are You? Honor Your Hunger

Lorena Keen

TABLE OF CONTENTS

INTRODUCTION

If you could trade out each diet like a frequent flyer program, the vast majority of us would have earned a free trip to the moon and back. The about $60 billion per year weight loss industry could finance such a trip for a long time even unto future generations. Amusingly, we appear to have more regard for our expensive automobiles than for ourselves. If you took your vehicle to an auto repairman for normal check-ups, and after time and cash spent, the vehicle continued with its faults; you wouldn't be hard on yourself, right? However, regardless of the way that 90 to 95 per cent of all weight loss routines and diets perform below expectations —you will always blame yourself, not the diet! Is it accurate to say that it isn't unexpected that with a high disappointment rate for various weight loss and diet routines—we don't blame the dieting process?

At first, when we wandered into the world of private practice, we didn't have any acquaintance with one another. However, independently, every one of us had strikingly comparative encounters that made us re-examine how we work. This prompted an extensive change by the way we practice and years after; the fact was the driving force for this book. In spite of the fact that we rehearsed independently of one another, unconsciously, every one of us began by making a promise to maintain a strategic distance from the trap of working with weight control. We would not like to deal with an issue that was just set up to fail in the long run. Be that as it may, while we attempted to stay away from weight reduction programs, doctors continued referring their patients to us. Normally, their blood pressure or cholesterol was high.

Whatever their clinical issues were, weight reduction was believed to be the fastest route of treatment. Since we needed to support these patients, we set out on the weight reduction program with a promise to do it better than we had in the past; the major aim was that our patients would succeed. They would be among that little 5 to 10 per cent success ratio.

We created simple but healthy meal plans based on our patients' preferences, ways of life, and explicit needs. These plans depended on the broadly accepted "exchange system" regularly utilized for diabetic meal plans and weight control. We disclosed to them this

was not a diet routine, for even in those days, we realized weight control plans didn't work. We acknowledged that these meal plans were not low-calorie diets since patients could pick between chicken, turkey, fish, or lean meat. They could have a bagel, a biscuit, or toast. If they truly needed a treat, they could have one
(not five!). They could top off with "free snacks and food" aplenty, so they never needed to feel hungry.

We explained to them that if they had a craving for a specific food, they could feel free to eat it without feeling guilty. In any case, we likewise advised delicately, yet firmly, that adhering to their customized meal plans would assist them with accomplishing their goals. As the weeks passed by, our customers were anxious to please us and strictly followed their meal plans. We weighed them every week; eventually, they met their weight loss target. Regrettably, sometime later, we began getting calls from a good number of these same individuals explaining to us why they desperately needed our services again.

Some way or another, the weight had returned on. Their calls were apologetic and persuasive. For reasons unknown, they couldn't stay on track any longer. Perhaps they required somebody to monitor them. Perhaps they needed more restraint. Possibly they simply weren't any great at this type of thing, and unquestionably, they felt remorseful and discouraged. Regardless of the "disappointment," our patients put all the blames on themselves. They confided in us—we were the "incredible nutritionists" who had helped them shed pounds. Consequently, they had done something wrong, not us. As time went on, it turned out to be evident that something was exceptionally amiss with this weight loss approach.

The entirety of our well-meaning goals was just fortifying some extremely negative, self-destroying ideas that our patients had about themselves—that they didn't have discretion, they couldn't do it accordingly; they were awful or wrong. This prompted blame, blame, and more blames on themselves. At this point, we had both arrived at a defining moment in the manner we counseled. How would we be able to morally continue showing individuals things that appeared to be logically and nutritionally stable, yet activated such passionate upheaval?

However, then again, how might we disregard an aspect of treatment that could have such a significant impact on a patient's future wellbeing? As we battled with these issues, we started to investigate a portion of the well-known literature that recommended a 180-degree rotation from dieting. It proposed a method for eating that took into consideration all kinds of food choices, without respect for nutritional values. Our underlying responses were exceptionally skeptical, if not absolutely dismissing.

We responded with self-righteous resentment. How would we be able to, as nutritionists (registered dietitians), trained to take a look at the associations among nutrition and wellbeing, endorse a method for eating that appeared to dismiss the very establishment of our philosophy and knowledge? The battle line was drawn. The healthy meal plans were not helping individuals keep up lasting weight control, yet the "toss out nutrition approach" was a hazardous alternative.

The recommendation to overlook food and dismiss how the body feels because of eating "anything you desire" limits the regard for one's body, which is the gift of life. In the long run, we settled the contention by creating up the INTUITIVE EATING PROCESS. This book is a link between the developing anti-diet movement and the health community. While the anti-dieting movement counters dieting and hails accepting your body the way it is (fortunately), it frequently neglects to address health dangers. How would you reconcile junk diet issues and still eat healthy meals, while you are not dieting? We will reveal to you how in this book.

If you are like the vast majority of our customers, you are tired of dieting but then alarmed by eating too much. A good number of our clients are uncomfortable in their bodies—however, they don't have a clue how to change for the better. Intuitive Eating gives another method for eating that is ultimately stress-free and sound for your mind and body. It is a process that releases the shackles of abstaining from excessive food intake (which can just prompt hardship, resistance, and rebound weight gain). It implies returning to your underlying foundations—

confiding in your body and its signals. Intuitive Eating won't just change your association with food; it might completely change you.

We trust that Intuitive Eating will make a huge difference in your life—it has for our customers. Indeed, when our customers discovered that we were writing this book, they were ready to share some particular defining moments with you:

- "Make certain to reveal to them that If they have a craving, it can really end up being an incredible encounter, since they'll find out a lot about their contemplations and emotions, because of such cravings."

- "Disclose to them that taking an opportunity to check whether they're hungry doesn't imply that they can't eat if they find they're not hungry. It's only an opportunity to ensure that they're not eating on autopilot. If they need to eat in any case, they can!"

- "When I go to a session, I feel as though I'm heading off to see the priest for confession. That originates from every one of the occasions I used to go to the dietician, and I would need to disclose to him how I had trespassed after he had weighed me. This isn't originating from you, but the internal Food Police."

- "I feel like I'm out of jail. I'm free and not pondering about food all the time any longer."

- "At times, I blow up, because good food has lost its magic on my taste buds. Nothing tastes as good as it did when it was forbidden. I continued searching for the old rush that food used to give me until I understood that my excitement in life wasn't going to originate from my eating any longer."

- "With consent, comes a decision. Furthermore, settling on decisions dependent on what I need and not on what another person is letting me know, feels so empowering."

- "Subsequent to quitting any pretense of binging, I wound up feeling truly low a portion of the time and even angry at different occasions. I understood that the food was concealing my awful sentiments. Be that as it may, it was likewise concealing my positive sentiments. I'd preferably feel better and terrible rather than not feeling at all!"

- "When I perceived the amount I was utilizing dieting and eating to adapt to life, I understood that I needed to change a portion of the stress in my life If I at any point needed to relinquish food as a way of dealing with stress."

- "In some cases, I have hungry days, and on other days I feel full. It's so pleasant to eat all the more some of the time and not feel remorseful that I'm conflicting with some dieting plan."

- "I get so elated when I see food I used to limit. Presently I believe—it's free, it's there, and it's mine!"

- "I'm so happy you're writing this book; it will enable me to clarify what I'm doing. All I know is that it works!"

- "When I'm in the diet mood, I can't consider the genuine issues in my life."

- "This is simply the best I've at any point I have taken care of myself in my life."

MINDFUL EATING VERSUS INTUITIVE EATING—IS THERE A DIFFERENCE?

We very frequently utilize the expression "Mindful eating" since it has gotten generally utilized and practiced by many. The Center for Mindful Eating states that mindful eating incorporates:

- Allowing yourself to get mindful of the positive opportunities that are accessible through food preparation and utilization, by regarding your very own inner wisdom.
- Choosing to eat meals that are both satisfying to you and nourishing to your body, by utilizing every one of your senses to explore, enjoy, and taste.
- Acknowledging reactions to varieties of food (preferences, neutral, or aversions), without judgment.

Learning to know about physical hunger and satiety signs to control your choice to start eating and to quit eating. While Intuitive Eating incorporates the standards of careful eating, it likewise envelops a more extensive way of thinking, tending to the issues of intellectual distortions and emotional eating. It incorporates considering fulfillment to be a focal point in eating, physical action/development for feeling better, dismissing counting calories mindset, utilizing sustenance data without judgment, and regarding your body, paying little respect to how you feel about its shape. Intuitive Eating is a dynamic process that involves coordinating a broader philosophy of mind, body, and food. Let us show you strategic steps on how to be successful with Intuitive Eating.

CHAPTER ONE: WHAT KIND OF EATER ARE YOU?

Maybe you are still abstaining from excessive food intake and don't know it! There are numerous kinds of eating styles that are really unconscious types of dieting. A good number of our patients have said they were not on a diet—however, after looking into what and how they eat, they were all the while unconsciously dieting! Here's an example: Ted came on the grounds that he needed to lose weight and become fit. He said that in his fifty years of living, he had been on just four serious diet plans.

When scrutinizing the book titles in the workplace (impulsive overeating books, emotional eating books, dietary disorder books, etc.), he expressed, "You work with a lot of real dieting disorders ... well, I'm not one of those." Ted obviously didn't consider himself to be a dieter, only a cautious eater. However, it worked out that he was an oblivious dieter. In spite of the fact that Ted was not effectively dieting, he was under-eating to a level where he was almost passed out in the evening. The explanation—he had consistently been unhappy with his weight!

In the mornings, he would go for a serious bicycle ride for 60 minutes, get back home, and have a little breakfast. Lunch was generally serving of mixed greens with frosted tea (while this sounds solid, it's excessively low in starches). By mealtime, his body would scream for carbs and good food. Ted was in an extreme calorie shortage, yet in addition, he refused to take enough carbohydrates. Night times are transformed into a food fest! Ted had thought he had a "food volume" disorder with a solid sweet tooth. In all actuality, he had an unconscious diet mindset that naturally set off his late-night eating and sweet tooth cravings.

Alicia likewise was not a conscious dieter. She came in not to get in shape, but since she needed to build her energy level. During the earlier session, it turned out to be evident that she had complicated issues with food. So she was queried as to whether she had been dieting a great deal. She looked shocked. "How did you know that I've been on zillions of diets?"

While Alicia claimed to approve of her present weight, she was still at war with eating right; she didn't trust herself with making appropriate food choices. For reasons unknown, Alicia had been abstaining from excessive food intake since she was a child. In spite of the fact that she was not officially abstaining from excessive food intake, she held (and extended) a lot of food rules that almost deadened her capacity to eat normally. We see this constantly, the headache from dieting: keeping away from specific foods no matter what, feeling crazy the minute a "forbidden" food is eaten, feeling regretful when deliberate food rules are broken, (for example, "Thou shalt not eat after 6 P.M., etc. unconscious dieting generally happens as meticulous dietary patterns. There can be a barely recognizable difference between eating for dieting and healthy eating. Notice how even the frozen diets, for example, Lean Cuisine and Weight Watchers are putting their emphasis on wellbeing instead of a diet.

For whatever length of time that you are occupied with some type of dieting, you won't be free from food and stress. Regardless of whether you are a conscious or an oblivious dieter, the effects are comparative—the diet backfires impact. This is described by periods of cautious eating, "blowing-it," and paying retribution with all the more slimming down or extra-cautious eating. In this chapter, we will investigate the dieting/eating styles to help see where you are present. Afterward, you will meet the Intuitive Eater, and the Intuitive Eating style, the answer for living healthy without diets.

THE EATING PERSONALITIES

To assist you with explaining your eating style (or dieting), we have recognized the accompanying key classifications of eaters that show trademark eating designs: the Careful Eater, the Professional Dieter, and the Unconscious Eater. These eating characters are displayed in any event, when not formally dieting. It's conceivable to have more than one eating character, despite the fact that we see that there tends as a dominant trait.

Occasions in your life can likewise impact or move your eating character. For instance, one customer, a tax lawyer, was normally a Careful Eater; however, during charge season, he turned into the Chaotic Unconscious Eater. You may wind up, at times, having the eating qualities portrayed under the three core eating characters. Observe this, and if your eating personality exists in one of these domains more often than not, it very well may be a disorder. Peruse each eating personality and see which one best mirrors your eating style.

By understanding where you are present, it will get simpler to figure out how to turn into an Intuitive Eater. For instance, you may discover you have been occupied with a type of dieting and not have known about it. Or on the other hand, you may find qualities that unwittingly neutralize you.

THE CAREFUL EATER

Careful eaters are the individuals who will, in general, be cautious about what food they put into their bodies. Ted was a case of a Careful Eater (by day). Superficially Careful Eaters give off the impression of being "flawless" eaters.

They are exceptionally food conscious. They usually appear health and wellness conscious (honorable attributes respected and reinforced in our general public).

EATING STYLE.

There is a scope of food practices that the Careful Eater shows. At one point, the Careful Eater may worry over every piece of food permitted into the body. Grocery shopping trips are spent examining food labels. Eating out regularly implies cross-examining the waiter—what's in the food, how is the food prepared—and getting affirmations that the food is prepared explicitly to the Careful Eater's admiration (generally not one bit of oil or other fat utilized in cooking).

What's wrong with this mindset? Aren't label reading and emphatic café requesting in the wellbeing interests of certain individuals? Obviously! The difference, be that as it may, is the power of the cautiousness and the capacity to relinquish any blame with respect to your eating decision. Careful Eaters tend to under-eat in small portions and screen the quality of food eaten. The Careful Eater can burn through a large portion of their waking hours, arranging out the next healthy snack or meal, frequently worried over what to eat.

While the Careful Eater isn't officially on a diet regimen, their brain is—scrutinizing each "undesirable," greasy, or sugary food eaten. The Careful Eater can run the scarce difference between being truly keen on health and wellbeing, and eating cautiously for body image. Now and again, Careful Eater is guided by time or events. For instance, some Careful Eaters are fastidious during the weekdays, so they acquire their "eating right" to "eat lavishly" on the weekends or for an up and coming party. Be that as it may, ends of the week happen 104 days of the year—the overeating it can backfire with undesirable weight gain. Therefore, it's not strange for a Careful Eater to think about on a diet.

THE PROBLEM

There's nothing amiss with being keen on the health and well-being of your body. The issue happens in any case, when diligent eating, influences a sound association with food—and contrarily impacts your body. Cautious Eaters, take after a chronic dieter style. They may not eat fewer carbs, yet they examine each food for quality and quantity.

THE PROFESSIONAL DIETER

Professional dieters are simpler to recognize; they are always dieting. They have typically attempted the most recent commercial diet, diet book, or new weight reduction trick. Now and again, abstaining from excessive food intake happens through fasting, or "cutting back." Professional Dieters know a great deal about of food, calories, and "slimming down stunts," yet the explanation they are consistently starting another diet routine is that the first one never worked. Today, the Professional Dieter is likewise knowledgeable in checking sugar/carbohydrate grams.

EATING STYLE

Professional dieters likewise have cautious eating characteristics. The distinction, in any case, is that chronic dieters control each eating decision for the sake of getting in shape, not really for health reasons. When the dieter isn't formally on a diet, the person is generally pondering on how quickly he/she can get started with the next diet. She frequently awakens, trusting this will be a decent day—the fresh start.

While Professional Dieters have a ton of dieting information, it doesn't work well for them. It's not irregular for them to binge or takes part in Last Meal eating the minute a forbidden food is eaten. That is on the grounds that chronic dieters genuinely accept they won't eat such food anytime soon; for tomorrow, they diet, tomorrow they begin once again with a fresh start. Better eat now; it's the last possibility. Of course, the Professional Dieter gets disappointed at the worthlessness of the endless loop. Diet, get in shape, put on weight, irregular binges, and back to dieting.

THE PROBLEM

It's difficult to live along these lines. Slimming down makes it progressively hard to shed pounds, not to mention eating refreshingly. Chronic under-eating typically brings about indulging or occasional binges. For some Professional Dieters, the disappointment of getting in shape turns out to be escalated to the point that they may attempt laxatives, diuretics, and diet pills. What's more, because these "diet aids" don't work, they may attempt outrageous strategies, for example, ceaseless limiting, as anorexia nervosa, or purging, (for example, vomiting after a binge), like bulimia.

While anorexia and bulimia are multi-factorial and established in psychological disorders, a growing body of research has shown that chronic dieting is not uncommon with dieting disorders. One study specifically found that when weight watchers arrive at the age of fifteen years, they are multiple times as liable to experience the ill effects of a dietary issue as non-dieters.

THE UNCONSCIOUS EATER

The Unconscious Eater is frequently occupied with paired eating—which is eating and doing another action simultaneously, for example, sitting in front of the TV and eating, or reading, and eating. Due to the nuances and absence of mindfulness, it very well may be hard for an individual to recognize this eating character. There are numerous subtypes of unconscious eaters. The Chaotic Unconscious Eater frequently carries on with an over-planned life, excessively occupied, such a large number of activities. The disorderly eating style is heedless; anything that's accessible will be snatched—candy machine toll, inexpensive food, it'll all do.

Nutrition and diet are frequently essential to this individual—only not in the crucial point in time of the chaos. Chaotic Eaters are regularly so bustling, putting out flames that they experience issues recognizing natural hunger until it's furiously insatiable. Of course, the unconscious eater goes on long stretches of time without eating. The Unconscious Eater is helpless against the insignificant nearness of food in any case if very hungry or full. Sweet jolts, food lying around at gatherings, food sitting on a kitchen counter—none will, for the most part, be left behind by the unconscious Eater. More often than not, in any case, the Unconscious eater doesn't know that they are eating, or the amount they are eating. For instance, the Unconscious Eater may cull up a few confections while in transit to the bathroom without monitoring it.

Social trips that rotate around food, for example, mixed drink parties and occasion buffets, are particularly extreme for the Unconscious Eater. The Unconscious Eater values every dollar used in eating. Their eating drive is frequently impacted by getting as much as they can for the cash.

The Emotional Unconscious Eater utilizes food to adapt to feelings, particularly awkward feelings, for example, stress, outrage, and dejection. While Emotional Eaters see their eating as the issue, it's regularly a side effect of a more profound issue. Eating practices of the Emotional Eater can go from snatching a sweet treat in stressful conditions to chronic compulsive binges of tremendous amounts of food.

THE PROBLEM

Unconscious eating in its different structures is an issue if it brings about constant indulging (which can easily happen when you are eating and not exactly mindful of it). Remember that somewhere close to the first and last nibble of food is the place the slip by of consciousness happens. As in, "Gracious, it's everything gone!" For instance, have you at any point purchased a huge box of sweets at the motion pictures and started to eat it just to find your fingers all of a sudden scratching the base of the unfilled box? That is a basic type of unconscious eating.

Yet, unconscious eating can likewise exist at a serious level, to some degree, modified condition of eating. For this situation, the individual doesn't know about what is being eaten, why he began eating, or even how the food tastes. This is daydreaming with food.

WHEN YOUR EATING PERSONALITY WORKS AGAINST YOU

In the end, the eating styles of the Careful Eater, the Professional Dieter, and the Unconscious Eater become an inadequate method for eating, in any event, when superficially, they show up OK. The answer to the frustrated eater: Try harder with another eating routine! From the start, the new diet appears to be elating and hopeful, however inevitably the natural weight gain returns. Abstaining from excessive food intake gets progressively troublesome, and in any event, when you continue your gauge eating character, it might feel more awkward than before.

This is on the grounds that with each diet, the internal food rules get more grounded. These foods frequently propagate sentiments of blame about eating in any event, when you are not officially abstaining from excessive food intake (dieting). Likewise, the organic impacts of dieting make it progressively hard to have an ordinary association with food. The Intuitive Eater character, be that as it may, is the special exception. It is the one eating style that doesn't work against your health and can assist you with chronic dieting and weight fluctuations.

INTRODUCING THE INTUITIVE EATER

Intuitive Eaters walk to their inward craving sign and eat whatever they pick without feeling guilt or any moral dilemma. The Intuitive Eater is an unaffected eater. However, it is very hard to be an unaffected eater in the present health-conscious society when you think about the types of food, and weight loss messages from ads, media, food professionals, and health experts.

Whenever we portrayed the basic eating characteristics of the Intuitive Eater to our customers, it's astonishing how regularly we'll hear the reaction, "That is how my husband eats." or "That is how my girlfriend eats." When we ask how that individual's weight and relationship to food are, the reaction is "zero issues!"

Consider babies. They are the natural Intuitive Eaters—basically free from cultural messages about food and self-perception. Babies have intrinsic knowledge of food. If you don't meddle with it, they don't eat dependent on abstaining from excessive food intake rules or health, yet various studies have shown that If you let a little child eat spontaneously, he will eat what he needs when given free access to quality meals. (This is presumably the hardest thing for a concerned parent to do—to let go and believe that children have an inborn capacity to eat!).

A milestone study, led by Leann Birch, Ph.D., published in the New England Journal of Medicine affirmed that preschool-age kids have a natural capacity to direct their eating as per what their body's requirement for development. This remains constant, with every meal, the little children's eating seems, by all accounts, to be a parent's bad dream. Researchers have found out that at a given meal, caloric intake was an exceptionally factor; however, it balanced out after some time. However, numerous guardians expect that their little youngsters can't manage their food consumption. Therefore, parents frequently embrace coercive systems trying to guarantee that the youngster eats healthy nutrition suitable for a growing child. In any case, past research by Birch and her partners demonstrates that such control strategies are counterproductive.

Besides, Birch notes that "guardians' endeavors to control their youngster's eating were accounted for more regularly by obese grown-ups than by grown-ups of normal weight." Similarly, Duke University analyst, Philip Costanzo, Ph.D., found that abundance weight in school-age kids was exceptionally connected with how much guardians attempted to limit their kids' eating. Indeed, even benevolent guardians meddle with Intuitive Eating. When a parent attempts to overrule a kid's regular eating signs, the tissue deteriorates, instead of getting better. A parent who provides food for a child at whatever point a craving signal is heard and who quits encouraging when the child shows that he's had enough can assume a powerful role in the initial development of Intuitive Eating.

Actually, notable work by specialist and dietitian Ellyn Satter has demonstrated that if you get the parents of overweight children to back off and give them a chance to eat without parental pressure, the children will, in the end, eat less than necessary. Why? The child starts to hear and comprehend his own inward signals of craving and satiety. The youngster additionally realizes that the individual will need to access food. As indicated by Satter, "Kids denied food trying to be thinly gotten distracted with food, apprehensive they won't get enough to eat and are inclined to binge when they find the opportunity." We have seen this as valid for grown-up dieters too. Only for grown-ups, the Intuitive Eating process has been covered for quite a while, regularly a long time.

Rather than having a parent slacken up the pressure, this relaxing of weight needs to originate from inside and against society's fantasy of dieting and distorted body worship. Luckily, we all have the characteristic Intuitive Eating capacity; it's simply been suppressed, particularly by regular dieting. This book is dedicated to telling you the best way to stir the Intuitive Eater within you!

HOW YOUR INTUITIVE EATER GETS BURIED

As babies get somewhat older, the mixed messages start to sneak in—from the early impacts of the Saturday morning commercial to the good-natured parent who cajoles his youngster to "Clean your plate." The coercion doesn't stop when you are a kid. There are a few external powers that impact our eating, which can additionally bury Intuitive Eating.

DIETING

You have just observed the harm that chronic dieting plays, including however not constrained to:

- Increased binge-eating
- Decreased metabolic rate
- Increased distraction with food
- Increased sentiments of deprivation
- Increased feeling of disappointment
- Decreased feeling of self-discipline

This serves to erode your trust with food and urges you to depend on outside sources to direct your eating patterns (a meal plan, a diet, the hour of the day, food rules, etc.). The more you go to outside sources to "judge" if your eating is under wraps, the further away you are from becoming an Intuitive Eater. Intuitive Eating depends on your inner prompts and signals.

EAT HEALTHY-OR-DIE MESSAGES.

Messages about eating healthily are all over, from philanthropic health organizations to food companies touting the medical advantages of their particular item. The innate message? What you eat can improve your wellbeing. On the other hand, take one wrong move (nibble), and you're one bit nearer to the grave. Is this an exaggeration? No. For instance, a 1994 official statement released by the Harvard School of Public Health expressed that eating trans-unsaturated fats (found in margarine) may cause thirty thousand deaths every year in the U.S. from coronary illness. That sort of message can easily leave you feeling remorseful for eating "an inappropriate" sort of food and feeling confounded about what you ought to eat.

Magazines and papers have additionally significantly expanded their inclusion of nutrition and wellbeing. One food editorial manager, Joe Crea, of a significant metropolitan paper, the Orange County Register (California), noticed that in a six-year time frame (1987–1993), his accounts on nutrition increased fivefold. Of about 800 nutrition stories, 200 were on health-related issues. While there is no uncertainty that what you eat can affect your wellbeing, the exponential media inclusion has filled in as a course to building nutrition distrustfulness in the buyer, particularly the dieter.

Joe Crea agrees, "You open the paper, see a wonderful lead story about cheesecake, and at the same time, another piece on how indulging in it will make you fat. It places the confusion in strife." Are we saying that you ought to overlook the virtues of healthy eating? Of course not. Nonetheless, when you have a “weight loss” mindset, the torrent of "good dieting" messages can make you feel guiltier about the food you decide to eat.

Obesity and Health announced a study on 2,075 grown-ups in Florida that uncovered that 45 percent of grown-ups felt regretful in the wake of eating foods they like. Women might be particularly guilt-ridden. An American Dietetic Association survey demonstrated that ladies feel guiltier than men about the food they eat (44 percent versus 28 percent). Could this be on the grounds that ladies' diet more as often as possible than men? Or then again, maybe ladies are normally the objective of health messages and food advertisements (think about the number of ladies' magazines).

Ladies are the key leaders for the family's health and nutrition planning, and are typically the watchmen of food and nutrition issues; also; they fill in as a practical objective. We have discovered that setting up food or good dieting as an underlying need in the Intuitive Eating process is counterproductive. To start with, we disregard nutrition, since it meddles with the way toward relearning how to turn into an Intuitive Eater. Nutrition heresy? No. It's conceivable to regard and respect quality food choices. It can't be the principal need when you've been dieting for your entire life. Or then again take a look at it along these lines; If you have concentrated all your thoughts on dieting, has it made any significant difference? The most nutritious eating plan (absolute) can be embraced as another type of dieting. The rest of this book will tell you bit by bit the best way to turn into an Intuitive Eater.

CHAPTER TWO: AROUSING THE INTUITIVE EATER: STAGES

The journey to Intuitive Eating resembles taking a cross-country trip. Before you even lash on your climbing boots, you need to realize what's in for your store during your adventure. While a guide is useful, it doesn't portray what you'll have to know to be sufficiently prepared, for example, trail conditions, atmosphere, uncommon touring spots, what sort of clothes to wear, etc. The motivation behind this section is to enable you to comprehend what's in store during your voyage to Intuitive Eating.

Regardless of whether it's climbing or relearning an all the more fulfilling eating style, you will experience numerous phases en route. The measure of time that you have to remain in a specific stage is variable and profoundly individualized. For instance, crossing new hiking trails relies upon how physically fit you are, the manner by which you manage dread of new trails, how much time you need to climb, and the accessibility of climbing trails. Essentially, your adventure back to Intuitive Eating relies upon to what extent you've been dieting, how emphatically entrenched in your diet thinking is, to what extent you've been utilizing food to adapt to life, that you are so ready to confide in yourself, and that you are so ready to make weight reduction an optional objective and figuring out how to turn into an Intuitive Eater the essential objective.

Here and there, you'll move to and fro within the stages. If you acknowledge this is a normal part of the process, it will assist you to keep going without feeling that you are breaking faith or not gaining ground.
Think about this situation: You are on a hiking trail and experience a byway that is difficult to interpret with your trail map. Do you go to one side or left? You contemplate for some time and choose to go left. While strolling, you spot something you've never observed, a splendid green caterpillar shimmying up a purple blossom. A couple of steps ahead, you find an unusual bird. In any case, a couple of steps past these wonders of nature is a major rock flagging that you picked an inappropriate way. You pivot, return to the fork, and take the other way. Was this alternate route an exercise in futility? No. Thus, on the way to Intuitive Eating, you will take many turns and examination with new musings and practices.

Intuitive Eating is altogether different from dieting. Dieters generally get disappointed when they don't pursue the eating regimen way precisely as recommended. We have seen numerous chronic dieters simply go astray at one meal, be critical for that error, and "blow" the eating regimen for that day or weekend or significantly more! Remember that the journey to Intuitive Eating is a process complete with high points and low points, in contrast to dieting when the regular desire is straight progress (losing a specific measure of weight in a particular time span).

The way to Intuitive Eating resembles "investing in a long-term mutual fund." After some time, there will be a return on the interest regardless of the day by day fluctuations of the securities exchange. Such should be normal and anticipated. How amusing that we have been instructed in economic matters, the everyday changes in the securities exchange are typical, and there is rarely a speedy get-rich fix, yet in the weight reduction business, "get slim quick" is regularly observed as the main objective for success.

Remember Webster's meaning of process: "a continued improvement involving numerous changes," and "a specific strategy for accomplishing something, by and large including various operations or activities." As with any process, it's essential to remain centered in the present and develop from the numerous encounters you will experience. Assuming; nonetheless, you focus on the final product (which for a great many people is the number of calories or pounds lost), it can make you feel discouraged and overwhelmed and winded up disrupting the process. Rather, If you recognize little changes en route and value the learning process (which can be stressful), it will assist you with remaining on the Intuitive Eating way and push ahead. When you really become an Intuitive Eater, your body will come back to its regular weight ' level and stay there. For some individuals, that implies shedding pounds.

To see whether you are a good candidate for weight reduction, ask yourself these questions:

- Have you routinely eaten past your agreeable fullness level?
- Do you routinely indulge when you're preparing for your next diet (knowing there will be a lot of meals you won't be permitted to eat)?

- Do you indulge as a method for dealing with stress in troublesome occasions or to top off time when you're exhausted?
- Have you likewise been impervious to work out?
- Do you possibly practice when you diet?
- Do you skip suppers or stand by to eat until you're eagerly very hungry, possibly to find that you indulge when you at long last eat?
- Do you feel regretful, either when you binge or when you eat an "a wrong meal," which brings about all the more indulging?

If you answered "yes" to a few or all of these inquiries, then, all things considered, you will have the luck to come back to your natural healthy weight after this process. When you've quit any pretense of slimming down perpetually, you'll end up eating far less food and needing to practice consistently. You'll see that your body feels so much better when your stomach isn't overloaded when your muscles are conditioned, and your heart is fit.

If you focus on how you feel like the objective, instead of on weight reduction, you'll find, unexpectedly, that you can't resist the urge to get in shape, rather, you will keep on concentrating on weight reduction as the objective, you'll get tied up in the old eating routine mindset thinking and searching for that perfect weight reduction resembling a carrot dangling on that stick before you—you're always dieting without being successful. Throughout the years, we have seen that our patients experience a five-step movement in figuring out how to become Intuitive Eaters.

The next section will assist you with getting a thought of what's in store on your personal journey to intuitive eating.

STAGE ONE: READINESS—HITTING DIET BOTTOM

This is the point many people start. You are painfully mindful that each endeavor to get in shape has ended in disappointment. You are burnt out on valuing every day, depending on whether the scale is up or down a pound or two (or If you've overeaten the day preceding). You think about food constantly. You talk about the unhealthy and restrictive food talk—"If only I didn't need to watch my weight, I could eat that," or "I had two snacks—I was quite awful at my weight game today."

Your weight could can be categorized as one of three examples: It's higher than any time in recent times; you are stuck at a level, and the pounds won't shed; or while not significantly overweight, you pick up and lose five or ten pounds as much of the time and quickly as your clothing gets grimy and afterwards clean once more. You have put some distance between biological appetite and satiety signals. You have overlooked what you truly prefer to eat and rather eat what you figure you "should" eat. Your association with food has built up a negative tone, and you fear eating the meals you love since you're might be difficult to stop.

When you surrender to the temptation of the "forbidden foods," it's not surprising to binge since you already feel regretful. However, you earnestly promise you will never eat them again. It's not uncommon to find that you eat to comfort, occupy, or even numb yourself from your emotions. If that is the situation, you will detect that a mind-blowing quality of life has been truncated by obsessive thoughts about food and by thoughtless eating. You already developed a negative opinion about your body image—you don't care for the manner in which you look and feel in your body, and your sense of pride is diminished. You have gained from your own experience that slimming down doesn't work—you have wound up in a sorry situation and feel stuck, baffled, and disheartened.

This stage continues until you conclude that you are troubled eating and living along these lines—and you are prepared to take care of business. Your first considerations may veer toward finding another eating routine to take care of your issues. Be that as it may, very quickly, you understand that you can't do that one until the end of time. If this is the place, you get yourself, at that point, you are prepared for the procedure that will take you back to eating naturally.

STAGE TWO: EXPLORATION—CONSCIOUS LEARNING AND PURSUIT OF PLEASURE

This is a phase of discovery and exploration. You will experience a period of hyper consciousness to help reacquaint yourself with your Intuitive sign: hunger, taste inclinations, and satiety. This stage is a lot, like figuring out how to drive a vehicle. For the new driver, simply getting the vehicle out of the carport requires

a lot of conscious deductions, complete with a psychological checklist:
Put the key in the start, ensure the gear is in park gear or neutral, turn on the ignition, check the rearview mirror, remove the hand brake, etc. This hyper consciousness is important to secure the entirety of the means required just to get that vehicle in first gear! In a similar sense, you will focus in on the details of eating that have advanced without such focused reasoning (Be that as it may, this is important to discover the Intuitive Eater in you). It might appear to be cumbersome and awkward, even over the top.

In any case, hyper consciousness is unique in relation to over the top reasoning. Fanatical believing is inescapable and is described by stress. It fills your psyche during the day and shields you from considering anything else. Hyperconsciousness is more explicit. It zooms in when you have an idea about food, however, leaves when the eating experience is finished. Also, much the same as the means required to drive a vehicle become autopilot for the experienced driver; Intuitive Eating will, in the long run, be experienced without this underlying awkwardness. You may feel that you are in a hyperconscious state for a significant part of the time during this stage. This may feel awkward from the outset and maybe even weird. Keep in mind, a lot of your past eating was either for the most part, oblivious or diet-coordinated.

In this stage, you'll start to make peace with food by giving yourself unrestricted permission to eat. This part may feel alarming, and you may decide to move gradually (within your comfort zone). You will figure out how to dispose of guilt-induced eating and start to find the significance of the fulfillment factor with food.

The more fulfilled you are when eating, the' less you will consider food when you are not hungry—you will never again be lurking in the shadows. You will try different things with foods that you have not eaten for quite a while. This incorporates dealing with your actual food of different preferences. You may even find that you don't care for the flavor of a portion of the foods you've been longing for! (Remember that long periods of counting calories, or eating what you "should," just serve to separate you from your inside eating drive and genuine food inclinations).

You will figure out how to respect your appetite and understand your body signals that show the numerous degrees of craving. You will figure out how to isolate these natural signs from the enthusiastic sign that may likewise trigger eating. In this stage, you may find that you are eating larger amounts of foods than your body needs. It will be hard to regard your completion at this stage since you need time to explore different avenues regarding the amount it takes to fulfill a denied sense of taste. It likewise requires some investment for you to create trust with food again and realize that it's genuinely alright to eat.

How might you respect fullness if you are not totally sure it's alright to eat a specific food, or If you dread it won't be there tomorrow? During this stage, weight gain normally stops or is constrained to only a few pounds. If you have been utilizing food emotionally, you may find that you will start to feel your emotions and may encounter distress, trouble, or even sorrow now and again. The greater part of your eating might be in foods that are heavier in fat and sugar than you've been familiar with—despite the fact that you may have been eating huge amounts of these foods unintentionally or with guilt. The manner in which you eat during this stage won't be the example that you will set up or need for a lifetime. You will see that your wholesome parity is unbalanced, and you may not feel physically in control during this time.

This is all normal and anticipated. You should release yourself through this phase for whatever length of time that you need. Keep in mind; you are compensating for a considerable length of time of hardship, negative self-talk, and blame. You are modifying positive food encounters, similar to a strand of pearls. Every food experience, similar to each pearl, may appear to be irrelevant, yet on the whole, they have any kind of effect.

STAGE THREE: CRYSTALLIZATION

In this stage, you will encounter the first arousals of the Intuitive Eating style that has consistently been a part of you, yet was covered under the thought of dieting. When you enter this stage, a significant part of the investigation work from the past stage starts to solidify and feels like big conduct change. Your considerations about foods are never again excessive. You barely need to keep up the hyper consciousness about eating that was initially required. Therefore, your eating choices don't require a lot of coordinated ideas. Rather, you find that your meal decisions and reactions to biological signals are primarily intuitive.

You have a more prominent feeling of trust—both in your entitlement to pick what you truly want to eat and in the way that your biological signals are reliable. You are more comfortable with your food decisions and will begin to enjoy true fulfillment at your mealtimes. Now, you respect your craving more often than before, and it's simpler to observe what you want to eat when you are hungry. You keep on making peace with food. What feels new in this stage is that it's simpler to stop amidst your meal to intentionally measure how much of your stomach is filling up.

You will be able to understand when you are full and regard the presence of that signal, despite the fact that you may find that you regularly eat past the fullness mark. The same principle applies for when an archer focuses on another objective; it regularly requires shooting numerous arrows before figuring out how to hit the bull's eye. You may be picking heavier foods more often than not, yet you will find that you don't require as quite a bit of them to fulfill you.

If you've been an emotional eater, you'll become very proficient at isolating biological hunger signals from emotional hunger. In view of this clarity, as a rule, you will encounter your feelings and discovering approaches to comfort and occupy yourself without the utilization of food. Some weight reduction may happen during this stage, particularly if you have a lot of weight to lose. If not, you'll see that you're keeping up your weight, instead of dealing with weight issues here and there. However, more significant than weight reduction at this stage is the feeling of prosperity and strengthening that starts to happen. You won't feel powerless and miserable any longer. You will start to regard your body and comprehend that it is the place it's at because of the dieting attitude, as opposed to the absence of self-discipline.

STAGE FOUR: THE INTUITIVE EATER AWAKENS

When you arrive at this stage, all the work you have been doing comes full circle in an agreeable, free-flowing eating style. You reliably pick what you truly need to eat when you are eager. Since you realize that you can have more food, based on your personal preference, at whatever point you are hungry, it's anything but difficult to quit eating when you feel easily full. You will start to find that you pick lighter and more beneficial foods, not on the grounds that you figure you should, but since you feel better physically when you eat along these lines. The dire need to demonstrate to yourself that you can have heavier foods will have decreased. You genuinely know and trust that these once illegal foods will consistently be there, and if you truly need to eat them, you can—so they lose their charming quality.

Chocolate begins to take on a similar emotional undertone as a peach. You won't have to test yourself any longer, and your deprivation troubles will be no more. When you do pick heavier foods, you will get extraordinary delight, and feel happy with a lot littler amount than any time in recent memory, and without guilt.

If adapting to your emotions has been hard for you, you will be less reluctant to encounter them and become progressively capable of sitting with them. Finding solid choices to divert and comfort yourself when fundamental will get normal for you. Your certain talk and self-talk will be certain and non-judgmental. Your peace agreement with food is immovably settled, and you will have discharged any contention or left-over blame about food decisions that you have conveyed. You will have quit being furious with your body and making disrespectful remarks about it. You will regard it and acknowledge that there is a wide range of sizes and shapes on the planet. Now, weight reduction will turn out to be progressively obvious, and your body will be en route to moving toward its common weight.

STAGE FIVE: THE FINAL STAGE—TREASURE THE PLEASURE

Now, your Intuitive Eater has been recovered. You will confide in your body's Intuitive capacities—it will be anything but difficult to respect your appetite and regard your completion. At last, you will feel no blame about your food decisions or amounts. Since you like your relationship to food and fortune, the delight that eating presently gives you, you will dispose of uninspiring eating circumstances and unappealing food sources. You will need to encounter eating in the most ideal of conditions and not pollute it with emotional stress. You will feel an inward conviction to quit any pretense of utilizing food to adapt to enthusiastic circumstances if that has been your habit. You will find that you would much rather manage your sentiments or occupy yourself from them with something besides food when feelings become excessively overpowering.

Since your eating style has become a wellspring of joy instead of a source of worry, you will see nutrition and exercise in a new way. The weight of the exercise activity will be lifted, and practicing will start to look alluring to you. Exercise will never again be utilized as the main impetus to consume more calories; rather, you become resolved to practice as an approach to feel much improved, physically, and rationally.
Similarly, quality nutrition will never again be another system for making you feel terrible about the manner in which you eat; rather, it turns into a way to feel as physically great and sound as you can. When you arrive at the last stage, your weight will normally diminish (If you had weight to lose) to a spot that is comfortable and fitting for your stature. If your weight was at that point normal, you would find that you can keep up it with no exertion and will be freed of the emotional good and bad times that go with the

restriction/binging cycles. Finally, you will feel engaged and shielded from external powers revealing to you what and the amount to eat, and how your body should look. You will feel free of the weight of counting calories. Furthermore, you will become an Intuitive Eater in every respect!

YOU CAN DO IT!

These stages and the progressions that happen with your eating and thoughts may appear to be unimaginable. Or on the other hand, they may appear to be excessively scary to follow through. For instance, the idea of giving yourself unending permission to eat may appear to be startling—and you may expect that you will never quit eating and will put on more weight. The rest of this book clarifies in extraordinary detail how to actualize every guideline, why it is required, and the basis behind it. You will likewise discover how other chronic dieters became Intuitive Eaters and how it transformed them. When you are done reading this book, you will realize that you also can turn into an Intuitive Eater and stop the madness associated with dieting.

CHAPTER THREE: REJECT THE DIET MENTALITY

Toss out the diet books and magazine articles that offer you the false teachings for getting thinner rapidly, effectively, and for all time. Reject at the falsehoods that have driven you to feel as though you were a disappointment each time a new a diet quit working for you, and you regained the entirety of the lost weight. If you permit even one little hope to believe that another and better diet may be hiding around the corner, it will keep you from allowing yourself to rediscover Intuitive Eating.

In case you're like most customers we see, the possibility of not dieting can be terrifying, in any event, when you realize that you can't force down one more diet plan or drink. It's entirely expected to feel panicky about relinquishing dieting, particularly when everyone around you is on some diet. It has been the main instrument you have known to get more fit, though briefly.

Winding up in a real diet, the predicament is a paralyzing feeling— one where you are doomed. If you diet and accursed if you don't. A good number of our customers feel stuck between these two clashing feelings of fear: "If I keep dieting, I'll ruin my digestion and put on weight," and "If I quit dieting, I'll put on more weight." Other normal apprehensions that we hear are:

FEAR: If I quit dieting, I won't quit eating.
REALITY: Dieting regularly triggers indulging.
Obviously, it's difficult to quit eating when you've been under-eating and restricting good nutrition; it's an ordinary reaction to starvation. But once your body learns, and believes, that you won't starve it any longer through dieting, the extreme drive for eating will diminish.

FEAR: I don't have a clue about how to eat when I'm not dieting.
REALITY: In case you're similar to most customers we see, the possibility of not dieting can be alarming, in any event, when you realize that you can't force down one more diet plan or drink. It's entirely expected to feel panicky about relinquishing abstaining from excessive food intake, particularly when your general surroundings is on some diet. It has been the main device you have known to get more fit, yet briefly. Winding up in a sorry situation is an incapacitating

inclination—cursed if your diet and condemned If you don't. Huge numbers of our customers feel stuck between two clashing feelings of fear: "If I keep dieting, I'll ruin my digestion and put on weight," and "If I quit slimming down, I'll put on more weight." Other regular apprehensions that we hear are:

FEAR: If I quit dieting, I won't quit eating.
REALITY: Dieting frequently triggers binging. Obviously, it's difficult to quit eating when you've been under-eating and limiting food; it's an ordinary reaction to starvation. (You'll hear increasingly about that in the following section!) But once your body learns, and believes, that you won't starve it any longer through dieting, the extraordinary drive for eating will diminish.

FEAR: I don't have the foggiest idea of how to eat when I'm not dieting.
REALITY: When you exile abstains from food and become an Intuitive Eater, you will eat in light of an inward flag, which will manage your eating. This resembles figuring out how to swim just because. The feeling of being surrounded by water can be unnerving to the beginner swimmer, particularly when

completely submerged. Likewise, being encompassed by food can be startling to the interminable dieter, who is figuring out how to eat once more. Yet, you won't figure out how to swim by simply remaining at the edge of the pool (even while accepting that figuring out how to swim is something worth being thankful for). First, you start by considering going all in and figuring out how to take in the water. In the end, you will place your head in the water when you are prepared—and you get increasingly agreeable.

FEAR: I will be out of control.
REALITY: You will feel in charge through Intuitive Eating, as opposed to depending on external factors and authority figures that you will undoubtedly resist. You will figure out how to tune in to and respect your inward signs, both physical and passionate—an incredible capacity.

THE DIET VOID

For some individuals', dieting has been an approach to adapt to life, from time to practicing a similarity to control. Think about the occasions throughout your life in which you started a diet. How regularly did your dieting harmonize with difficult transitions or moments? It's not bizarre to start a diet during the accompanying life transitions: going from childhood to adolescence, leaving home, and wedding, beginning a new job or encountering marital troubles. While counting calories may have been useless, it offered fervor and expectation—the invigoration of brisk weight reduction and the energy of watching the scale inch downwards, the expectation that this diet will be it. It's like setting off to a beautician for another cut, with the desire that it will alter the manner in which you look and feel about yourself and perhaps transform you. However, when you bid farewell to the rush and fervor of dieting, you'll likewise be relinquishing the bogus expectation and dissatisfactions from dieting.

There is a social component to dieting that you may miss, diet holding. When you choose to quit any pretense of abstaining from excessive food intake, you may be shocked how frequently new diets and dieting are the themes of discussion at parties, with companions, at work—and now you won't play that game. It may feel like an unquestionable requirement see motion picture everybody is discussing, just you haven't seen it and have no designs to see it either.

You may feel somewhat left out, isolated. Keep in mind, as long as there is cash to be made; there will consistently be another program or diet for a fast weight reduction fix.

PSEUDO-DIETING

A considerable lot of our customers state, "I've quit all forms of dieting," however they experience difficulty shaking off the diet attitude. They might be physical of a diet. However, the dieting contemplations remain. The issue is those dieting thoughts, as a rule, convert into a diet like practice, which becomes pseudo-dieting or oblivious abstaining from excessive food intake. So, these customers will, in any case, endure the symptoms of dieting, yet it's a lot harder to spot (and afterward they truly feel wild with their eating).

Pseudo-dieting practices are not typically obvious to the individual occupied with them. Remember that eating is universal, which makes it difficult to be objective. It very well may be hard to discover the loopholes in your eating mindset/conduct. If you don't have the foggiest idea of what you are searching for. To the shock of our customers, they frequently don't find that they have been pseudo-dieting until together we audit their eating history. Here are a few instances of pseudo-dieting :

- Meticulously checking sugar grams is the advanced adaptation of counting calories. While being aware of what you eat has its merits, the demonstration of checking starch grams to control weight is actually the same as counting calories. A considerable lot of our constant calorie counters are geniuses at rationing their starch grams for the afternoon—and they are trapped.

- Eating just "safe" foods. This typically implies staying with fat-free as well as low-calorie meals, beyond calculating fat grams. For instance, one customer would not eat any food that recorded more than one gram of fat on the food label, paying little attention to what her complete fat and calorie admission for the day was. Keep in mind, notwithstanding, that one meal, one snack, or one day won't represent the truth your health status or your weight.

- Eating just at specific times of the day, regardless of whether you are hungry, is a normal habit from dieting, particularly not eating following a specific time of night, for example, after 6:00 P.M.
- Reality: Our bodies don't punch clocks; we don't want all of a sudden, reduce our requirement for energy. This can particularly be an issue for a dieter who practices after work, returns home late—around 7:30 P.M.— and chooses it's past the point where it is possible to eat for fear that the fat meter is in high gear! While it is sensible not to have any desire to want to hit the bed on a full stomach, to deny a hungry body, any food or energy requirements is preposterous. Paying penance for eating "bad" foods, for example, treats, cheesecake, or frozen yogurt. The punishment can include skipping the next meal, eating less, vowing to be "great" tomorrow, or doing additional exercise.

- Cutting back on food, particularly when feeling fat or when a unique occasion, for example, a wedding or class get-together comes up. While cutting back sounds guiltless enough, it's stunning how frequently this gets carried on as oblivious under-eating. Keep in mind, under-eating as a rule triggers indulging.

- Pacifying hunger by drinking espresso or diet pop. This is a typical slimming down stunt to mollify food cravings without eating or calories.

- Limiting carbohydrates: We are struck by the number of customers who claim they are aware of the significance of devouring this fuel, yet eat a lacking measure of starches, for example, bread, pasta, and rice, since they are afraid they will put on weight.

- Putting on a "false food face" out in the open, eating just what is "legitimate" before other individuals. One customer, Alice, ate an agreeable meal with companions. When the treat plate came around, she truly needed a bit of pie, yet battled the desire since she needed to give off an impression of being a sound, chronic dieter. Be that as it may, on her way home, the desire for the pie expands into a wild hankering. Alice halted at the store, purchased an entire pie, and ate one-fourth of it, which was more than she would have eaten had she respected her actual food inclination before that moment!

- Competing with another person who is dieting — feeling committed to being similarly serious-minded (if not more). Since dieting is seen as a temperate characteristic in our general public, it isn't surprising that you would get sucked into seeming upright. This can easily happen when companions, family, or a noteworthy other is abstaining from excessive food intake.

- Second-speculating or passing judgment on what you have the right to eat depends on what you've eaten before in the day, as opposed to on hunger signals. One customer, Sally, ate two huge bowls of puffed rice grain for breakfast, subsequent to running for 60 minutes. She felt that was an excessive amount of food and, later in the midmorning, didn't enable herself to eat, in spite of the fact that she was hungry. Sally figured, "How might I be hungry just two hours after I had a major breakfast?" The truth for Sally was that while her volume of food toward the beginning of the day was bigger than her standard, it was as yet insufficient for the measure of activity she had done. Her body was attempting to advise her, "I need more fuel," yet Sally felt remorseful for being hungry. She additionally felt regretful for having a major breakfast, until she understood that in reality, she had under-eaten. Because a feast or bite doesn't fit the "standard" divide size from your dieting days, it doesn't mean you are indulging!

- Becoming a veggie-lover just to get thinner. A vegetarian's way of life can be a sound method for eating and living, yet If it is understood with a diet attitude, it turns out to be only another diet. For instance, Karen started eating meatless to get more fit. Yet, a month into her veggie lover eating, she started desiring meat. At no other time had she encountered meat desires! Karen acknowledged she never truly planned to turn into a veggie lover. She wasn't keen on veggie lover eating for wellbeing or moral issues, just as a vehicle to get more fit; thus, her eating regimen exploded backward.

THE DIETER'S DILEMMA

Whether you are occupied with genuine dieting or pseudo-dieting, any type of dieting will undoubtedly prompt issues. The Dieter's Dilemma is activated with the craving to be slim, which prompts abstaining from excessive food intake. That is the point at which the quandary unfurls. Dieting builds yearnings and inclinations for food. The dieter surrenders to the cravings indulge, and in the long run, regains any shed pounds. At that point, he has returned to where he began, at the first weight—or higher. What's more, by and by, the dieter wants to be thin; thus, another diet starts. The Dieter's Dilemma is propagated and deteriorates with each turn of the cycle. The dieter gets heavier and gets a handle on a greater amount of control with eating. How would you break the pointless Dieter's Dilemma? In spite of the fact that the anti-dieting development is developing in prominence, there is constantly another eating regimen or program around the corner. You should essentially settle on the choice to quit any form of dieting.

THE MOST EFFECTIVE METHOD TO REJECT THE DIET MENTALITY

To relinquish the dieting legend and the slimming down mentality, our minds require another frame of. In his best-seller book, The 7 Habits of Highly Effective People, writer Stephen Covey advanced the idea of how we see and understand the world around us. A paradigm is a model or reference by which we see and comprehend the world. In the realm of weight management, slimming down is the social paradigm by which we endeavor to control our weight.

A change in outlook is a break from the norm of cultures with old perspectives, with old ideal models. We should change our mindset to I refuse to diet; at exactly that point would we be able to construct a sound association with food and our bodies. While Covey's work is known in the business network, he hits upon an issue that sounds accurate for ceaseless dieters. He accepts that individuals are regularly attracted to cure the issue regardless of the long-term implications of this "handy solution." He feels that this methodology really worsens the issue instead of for all time understanding it. He identified the physical body like a prized resource that frequently is destroyed, while one is on the race for fast outcomes and transient advantages. Here are the means of starting your change in perspective and dismissing the diet mentality.

STEP I: RECOGNIZE AND ACKNOWLEDGE THE DAMAGE THAT DIETING CAUSES

There is a significant number of research on the health issues that are caused by dieting causes. Recognize that the damage is genuine, and that continued dieting will just worsen your issues. A portion of the key symptoms gathered from significant considers portrayed underneath in two classes, emotional and biological. As you read, take personal stock and inquire from yourself which of the issues you are as of now encountering. Knowing that dieting is the issue will assist you with getting through the wrong cultural myth that diets work. Keep in mind, if dieting is the issue, how might it be a piece of the grand solution?

HARM FROM DIETING: BIOLOGICAL AND HEALTH

In every century, starvation and human starvation has existed. Unfortunately, this is genuine even today. Survival of the fittest in the past meant survival of the fastest—just those with satisfactory energy stores (fat) could endure starvation. Therefore, our bodies are as yet prepared in this cutting edge age to battle starvation at the cell level. To the extent the body is concerned, dieting is a type of starvation, despite the fact that it's intentional. Constant slimming down has been appeared to:

- Teach the body to hold increasingly fat when you start eating once more. Low-calorie abstains from food twofold the catalysts that make and store fat in the body. This is a type of organic remuneration to enable the body to store more vitality, or fat, in the wake of dieting. Slow of weight reduction with each progressive endeavor to abstain from food. This has been demonstrated to be valid in both rodent and human studies.

- Decrease digestion - Dieting triggers the body to turn out to be progressively effective at using calories by bringing down the body's requirement for vitality

- Increase binges and cravings - The two people and rodents have been shown to indulge after chronic food restriction. Food restriction animates the mind to dispatch a course of desire to eat more. After significant weight reduction considers show that rodents lean toward eating progressively fat, while individuals have been appeared to incline toward foods both high in fat and sugar.

• Increase danger of premature death and coronary illness - A thirty-two year investigation of in excess of 3,000 people in the Framingham Heart Study has demonstrated that paying little respect to begin weight, individuals whose weight more than once goes here and there—known as weight cycling or dieting —have a higher generally speaking demise rate and double the typical danger of dying on from coronary illness. These outcomes were free of cardiovascular hazard factors and remained constant in any case if an individual was slim or stout. The harm from dieting might be equivalent to the dangers of remaining obese. Likewise, the results of the Harvard Alumni Health Study show that individuals who lose and gain at least eleven pounds within ten years, don't live as long as the individuals who keep up a steady weight.

• Satiety prompts atrophy - Weight watchers, for the most part, quit eating because of self-imposed limits as opposed to internal signals of fullness. This, joined with skipping meal s, can condition you to eat suppers of an increasingly bigger size.

• May cause body shape to change - Dieters who ceaselessly regain the shed pounds will, in general, regain weight around the stomach. This sort of fat stockpiling increases the danger of coronary illness. Other recorded reactions include cerebral pains, menstrual inconsistencies, weariness, dry skin, and male pattern baldness.

HARM FROM DIETING:

Psychological and Emotional Psychological specialists detailed the accompanying unfriendly impacts at the Landmark 1992 National Institutes of Health, Weight Loss and Control Conference:

- Dieting is connected to dietary problems.
- Dieting may cause pressure or make the dieter more helpless against its effects.
- Independent of body weight itself, dieting is connected with sentiments of disappointment, brought down confidence, and social uneasiness.
- The calorie counter is regularly powerless against loss of authority overeating while damaging "the

guidelines" of the diet, regardless of whether there was a genuine or seen offense of the eating regimen! The insignificant view of eating prohibited food, paying little mind to genuine calorie content, is sufficient to trigger indulging. In a different report, therapists David Garner and Susan Wooley present a convincing defense against the significant expense of bogus expectation from dieting.

They infer that:

- Dieting progressively disintegrates certainty and self-trust.
- Many large people accept they couldn't have become stout except if they had some principal character shortage. Gainer and Wooley contend that while numerous stout people may encounter gorging and sadness, these mental and social manifestations are the aftereffect of abstaining from excessive food intake. Be that as it may, these overweight people effectively decipher these side effects as additional proof of a basic issue. However, corpulent individuals don't have over the top mental unsettling influences contrasted with typical weight individuals.

STEP 2: BEWARE OF DIET-MINDSET TRAITS AND THINKING

The diet mindset surfaces in subtle forms when you choose to dismiss dieting. It's essential to perceive basic attributes of the eating regimen mindset; it will fill you in regarding whether you are as yet playing the dieting game. Disregard self-control, being respectful and failing.

DISREGARD WILLPOWER

While no specialist would anticipate that a patient should "will" circulatory strain to typical levels, doctors every now and again anticipate that their overweight patients should "will" their weight reduction by confining their food, as per Susan Z. Yanovski, M.D. This is likewise an overall frame of mind among our customers and numerous Americans—all you need is resolution and a little discretion.

In a 1993 Gallup survey, the most widely recognized impediment to getting more fit referred to by ladies was self-control. For instance, Marilyn is a successful legal advisor who moved to the highest point of the corporate ladder. She credits hard work, determination, and self-control as being liable for her prosperity. However, when she attempted to utilize these model standards in her dieting endeavors, she was terrible at it. Whatever achievement she had accomplished in her professional life was dulled by her feeling of disappointment with eating.

For what reason was Marilyn ready to be so taught in one part of her life, however, not in the other? "Discipline" is gotten from the word "disciple." According to Stephen Covey's work, if you are a follower of your very own profound qualities that have a superseding reason for existing, almost certainly, you'll have the will to complete them. Marilyn accepted profoundly that composing demanding agreements and keeping flawless records were imperatives to building certainty with her customers and her law office. However, some way or another, hearing that bread wasn't right on one diet, and anything with sugar wasn't right on another, didn't cause a similar sort of profound convictions.

Attempt as she may, she couldn't generally accept that chocolate chip treats were that underhanded! Self-discipline can be characterized as an endeavor to counter characteristic wants and supplant them with prescriptive principles. The longing for desserts is regular, ordinary, and very lovely! Any diet that lets you know, you can't have desserts is conflicting with your common want. The eating regimen turns into a lot of inflexible guidelines, and these sorts of rules can just trigger resistance. Self-control doesn't have a place in Intuitive Eating. As Marilyn turned into an Intuitive Eater, she found that tuning in to her own sign fortified her characteristic impulses, as opposed to battling them. She had nobody else's proscriptive principles to pursue or to oppose. Marilyn has quit taking on the apparition determination conflict, and she has lost all the weight with which she had been battling.

DISREGARD BEING OBEDIENT

A benevolent recommendation by a companion or huge other, for example, "Nectar, you ought to have the seared chicken "or "You shouldn't eat those fries" can set off an inward food resistance. In this kind of food battle, your solitary weapon to battle back turns into a twofold request of fries. Our customers call this overlook your eating. In material science, opposition consistently happens as a response to compelling. We see this rule in real life in the public arena—revolts frequently eject when the power of power turns out to be excessively incredible.

Additionally, the straightforward demonstration of being determined what to do (regardless of whether it's something you need to do) can trigger a defiant chain response. Much the same as "horrible two-year-olds or young people who revolt to demonstrate they are free, dieters can start defiant eating in the light of the demonstration of dieting, with its arrangement of unbending rules directing what to eat. As it's not astonishing to get notification from our customers that disrupting the guidelines of a diet makes them feel simply like they did when they were rebellious teenagers. In any case, cheer up, disobedience is an ordinary demonstration of self-safeguarding—securing your space or individual limits.

Think about an individual limit as a tall block fence encompassing you, with just one door. No one but you can open that door if you pick. Accordingly, nobody is permitted inside, except if you welcome the individual in. Inside your fence, live private emotions, considerations, and organic signals. Individuals who accept they realize what you need and instruct you are picking the lock to your door, or attacking your limits. Nobody might comprehend what's inside except if you let him know, by welcoming him in. What slims down or eat less advocate can know when you are hungry or what amount of food it will take to fulfill you?

In what capacity can anybody yet you know what surface and taste sensations will satisfy your sense of taste? In the realm of abstaining from excessive food intake, individual limits are crossed at numerous levels. For instance, you are determined what to eat, its amount to eat, and when to eat it. These choices should all be close to home decisions, with deference for singular independence and body signals. While food direction may originate from somewhere else, you ought to at last be liable for the when, what, and the amount of eating. When a nutritionist or diet attacks your limits, it's not unexpected to feel weak. The more you pursue the food limitations, the more prominent the attack on your self-governance. Here is the place the oddity lies. When abstaining from excessive food intake, you will probably revolt by eating more—to reestablish your independence and secure your limits. In any case, the demonstration of revolting can make you feel as wild as a city revolt.

Rather, you have an inward food battle on your hands. In any case, when the food insubordination is released, its force fortifies sentiments of the absence of control and the conviction that you don't have self-control. At last, you start to suffocate in an ocean of self-uncertainty and disgrace. What starts as mentally sound conduct, finishes in calamity. At last, weight reduction is undermined because of individual limit security. With Intuitive Eating, there is no compelling reason to revolt, since you become the one in control! Limits are additionally attacked when somebody makes remarks about your weight or how you should look. Once more, you will undoubtedly revolt by indulging. It's a method for saying "overlook you" by and by; "You reserve no option to disclose to me what to gauge."

DISREGARD FAILURE.

A lot of our dieting clients walk into our offices, feeling as though they are disappointments. Regardless of whether they are government officials, prominent big names, or straight-A students, they all discuss their food encounters disgracefully, and they question whether they'll ever have the option to feel successful in the area of eating. The dieting can trigger feelings of progress or disappointment. You can't come up short at Intuitive Eating—it's a learning process at each point along the way. What used to be thought of as a difficulty will rather be viewed as a growth experience. You'll get directly in the groove again when you see this as improvement, not disappointment.

STAGE 3: GET RID OF THE DIETER'S TOOLS

The dieter depends on external forces to control his eating, adhering to a controlled food plan, eating because it is the ideal time, or eating just a predetermined (and estimated) amount of food, regardless of whether they are hungry or not. The dieter additionally approves progress by external forces, essentially using the scale, asking, "What number of pounds have I lost? Is my weight up or down?" It's an ideal opportunity to toss out your dieting tools and books. Dispose of the meal plans and the bathroom scales. If all it took was a decent "reasonable" calorie-restricted meal plan to become fit, we would be a country of thin individuals—free meal plans are promptly accessible from magazines, papers, and even some food organizations.

THE SCALE AS FALSE IDOL

"If it's not too much trouble given the number a chance to be ... " This unrealistic number of prayers isn't happening in the gambling clubs of Las Vegas, yet in private homes all through the nation. In any case, much the same as the desperate gambler trusting that his fortunate number will come in, so is it worthless for the dieter to pay tribute to the "scale god." In one scope of the scale roulette, expectations and desperation make a daily dramatization that will, at last, shape what state of mind you'll be in for the afternoon. Incidentally, "good" and "bad" scale numbers can both trigger indulging—regardless of whether it's a salutary eating festivity or an encouragement party. The scale ritual undermines the body and mind endeavors; it can in one minute debase days, weeks, and even a very long time of dieting progress.

WHEN A POUND IS NOT A POUND

Numerous components can impact an individual's weight, which doesn't mirror the individual's ratio of muscle to fat. For instance, two cups of water gauge one pound. If you will, in general, hold water or swell, the scale can undoubtedly raise a couple of pounds without an adjustment in what you have eaten. However, for the oft coerce ridden dieter, the outcomes of water weight can appear to be extreme. For instance, we have had numerous patients feel terrible about eating an additional pastry throughout the end of the week and gauge themselves on the next Monday. The scale shoots up five pounds—and they accept they increased five pounds of fat.

Since lots of dieters are fast with the calorie calculator cruncher, we ask, "Did you eat an extra 17,500 calories throughout the end of the week?" obviously not, would be their answer. However, to make five pounds of fat requires a caloric overabundance of 17,500 calories better than average eating (one pound of fat is identical to 3,500 calories). So how would you clarify the weight gain?

WATER WEIGHT

Whenever the scale all of a sudden ascents or falls, it is normally a result of a liquid component in the body. Eating high-sodium foods can likewise incite water maintenance (not fat retention) in salt-touchy people. However, how effectively interminable dieters accept they accomplished something incorrectly; they should have without any assistance eaten five pounds worth of food! No! No! No! Likewise, shedding two pounds quickly from an hour of heart stimulating exercise is anything but a two-pound fat misfortune. Or maybe, it's generally water loss from sweat.

Happy dieters who imagine that they have shed ten pounds in seven days might be in for an undesirable shock. While the facts may confirm that the scale demonstrated ten pounds not as much as when they weighed days back, the real question is, what sort of weight did they lose? To shed ten pounds of fat in a week requires an energy loss of 35,000 calories or a deficiency of 5,000 calories every day! The normal lady just eats around 1,500 to 1,600 calories for each day.

The sad truth is that this individual is losing a ton of water weight, for the most part, to the detriment of their muscles, because of the process of muscle-wasting. Muscle is made up of the most part of water (around 70 percent). When a hungry body isn't given enough calories, the body rips apart itself for an energy source. The prime order of the body is that it must have vitality, at any cost—it's a piece of the endurance system. The protein in muscles is changed over to important vitality for the body. When a muscle cell is crushed, water is discharged, and in the long run, discharged—there's your valuable weight reduction.

The lost muscle adds to reducing your digestion. Muscles are metabolically dynamic tissue—(for the most part, the more muscle we have, the higher our metabolic rate.

That is one reason men consume a bigger number of calories than ladies—they have more bulk. Muscle additionally occupies less room than fat.

While this is positively valuable, a chronic dieter regularly gets baffled by the rising or constant scale number. The scale doesn't reflect body creation—simply like gauging a bit of steak at the butcher doesn't reveal to you how to fit the meat is. Saying something regarding the scale just serves to keep you concentrated on your weight; it doesn't help with the way toward getting back to reality with Intuitive Eating. Consistent weight checks can leave you baffled and hinder your progress. The best option—quit weighing yourself!

INTUITIVE EATING TOOLS

The instruments of the Intuitive Eater are inward signals, not outside powers revealing to you what, when, and the amount to eat. Yet, to acquire and comprehend these internal signals, you need another arrangement of intensity power tools—or rather, strengthening tools, which will be talked about in the following sections of this book.

CHAPTER FOUR: HONOR YOUR HUNGER

Keep your body sustained biologically with sufficient nutrients as well as carbohydrates. Else, you can trigger a basic drive to overeat. When you arrive at the point of excessive appetite, all aims of moderate, conscious eating are fleeting and irrelevant. Figuring out how to respect this first biological sign makes way for revamping trust with yourself and with food. A dieting body is a destitute body. Crazy comparison? No. While a dieting body may not resemble a starving individual in Ethiopia or Somalia, the "manifestations" from slimming down display a striking likeness to the starvation state.

The body doesn't have a clue about that there is a McDonald's everywhere as you set out on a diet. To the extent the body is concerned, it is living in a starvation state and needs to adjust. Our requirement for nutrients (energy) is so basic and base that if we are not getting enough vitality, our bodies normally repay with incredible biological and mental systems. The intensity of food restriction was distinctly exhibited in a landmark starvation study directed by

Dr. Ancel Keys during World War II, intended to help famine sufferers.

The subjects of the examination were thirty-two solid men who were chosen since they had predominant "psychobiological stamina"— prevalent mental and physical wellbeing. During the initial three months of the examination, the men ate; however, they wanted, 3,492 calories every day. The following a half year was the semi-starvation time frame. The men were required to lose 19 to 28 percent of their weight contingent upon their body creation. Calories were sliced almost down the middle, to a normal of 1,570 every day. The impacts of the semi-starvation were surprising, and strikingly reflect the side effects of chronic dieting :

- Metabolic rates diminished by 40 percent.
- The men were fixated on food. They had uplifted food longings and discussed food and gathering plans.
- The eating style changed—wavering from covetous swallowing to slowing down out the eating experience. A few men played with their food and tarried over a feast for two hours.

- The scientists noticed that "Few men neglected to hold fast to their eating regimens and revealed scenes of bulimia." One man was accounted for to have endured a total loss of "self-discipline" and ate a few treats, a sack of popcorn, and two bananas. Another subject, "outrageously defied the dietary guidelines," and ate a few sundaes and malted grains and even took penny treat.
- Some men practiced intentionally to acquire expanded food ^ proportions.
- Personalities changed, and as a rule, there was the beginning of lack of care, touchiness, irritability, and wretchedness. During the refeeding time frame, when the men were by and by permitted to eat freely, hunger got voracious. The men thought that it was hard to quit eating. The end of the week spends too much meant 8,000 to 10,000 calories. It took most of the men a normal of five months to standardize their eating. It's essential to recollect that during the time of these exemplary studies, there were no Arnold Schwarzeneggers or wellness and food divas. Sustenance inquires about what was simply in its earliest stages.

However, these men encountered a base fixation on food that was not media-driven or society-driven;

rather, it was activated by a natural endurance system.

Such conduct had never been seen in these men before their food hardship experience! Despite the fact that this is an exemplary starvation study, the caloric level is illustrative of a cutting edge weight reduction diet for men of 1,500 calories. These men were eating. Envision if a similar report was held under the present weights to be flimsy. We have had a few customers perused the exemplary Keys study, and they are struck by the comparability of their own encounters to those of the semi-starved men.

MECHANISM THAT TRIGGERS EATING

Regardless of whether you are a chronic dieter or not, amazing organic components are activated when your body doesn't get the vitality from food that it needs. It's no accident that food is incorporated as one of the basic human needs in Maslow's Hierarchy of Needs—a model that positions human needs, proposing that specific fundamental needs should be met before you can proceed to satisfy increasingly complex ones. Food and vitality are so basic to the endurance of the human species that if we don't eat enough, we set off a natural circuit that turns on our eating drive both physically and mentally.

The craving drive is genuinely a mind-body association. Eating is critical to such an extent that the nerve cells of hunger are situated in the nerve center of appetite located in the hypothalamus of the brain. A variety of biological signals trigger eating. What numerous individuals accept to be an issue of self-discipline is rather a natural drive. The power and force of the organic eating drive ought not to be thought little of. The neurochemicals from the mind coordinate our eating behavior with our body's natural need. Through an unpredictable arrangement of a compound and neural criticism, the mind screens the vitality needs of all our body frameworks, minute to minute. Furthermore, it makes decided compound orders concerning what we ought to eat. Fasting is especially dangerous to hunger control. It basically turns on the hormone switches on that initiate us to eat.

Numerous studies have demonstrated that bringing down body weight by food limitation and dieting has neither rhyme nor reason metabolically or to our mind science. Truth be told, it's counterproductive. The hormones that control craving likewise also influence dispositions and perspective, our physical vitality, and our sexual experiences. Most professionals concur that there are both complex biological and mental components that impact our eating. In this section, we will concentrate on the essential natural systems that turn on our longing to eat, particularly if we have denied our bodies of good food or dieting. There is increased digestion In starved people as studies have demonstrated that the body gets naturally prepared for the moment of eating, similar to a sprinter squatted in a prepared situation for a dangerous beginning, the minute the beginning gun is activated.

- Salivation increases with the increase of food deprivation, in any event, when there is no food present or proposal of eating! This has been shown in considers both on dieters and normal (non-dieting) people.
- Increased digestive hormones have been found in dieters both before and after eating.

THE CARBOHYDRATE CRAVER:

Neuropeptide Y

Neuropeptide Y (NPY) is a hormone produced by the cerebrum that triggers our drive to eat carbohydrates, the body's essential, and favored wellspring of vitality. While the majority of what we think about NPY originates from look into on rodents, there is a great deal of proof that shows that this mind synthetic can profoundly affect human eating conduct too by expanding both the size and term of starch-rich meals. Food deprivation or under-eating drives NPY without hesitation, making the body look for more carbohydrates. When the following meal or eating opportunity moves around, it can easily transform into a high-starch gorge—not on the grounds that you need determination or are crazy; it's your science (rather, NPY) shouting, "Feed me." NPY is fired up after any forced time of food deprivation, including a medium-term quick from meal to breakfast. NPY's levels are normally the most noteworthy in the first part of the day as a result of the momentary food deprivation from a medium-term quick.

The raised NPY levels are a part of the natural reason for eating early in the day! During an overnight fast, your body's stores of sugars in the liver are depleted and need topping off. You truly wake up on void in the first part of the day. Be that as it may, if you skip breakfast, you are probably going to pay for it with an increase in NPY level, which can lead to mid-evening time pigging out. The mind likewise makes more NPY when sugars are being used as fuel and in the midst of stress.

Eating carbohydrates reduce NPY through its impact on serotonin, another hormone in the brain. As we eat more starches, it builds the generation of serotonin, which thus stops the creation of NPY and puts an end to the desire for sugars. The more you deny your actual appetite and battle your characteristic science, the more grounded and increasingly serious food yearnings and cravings become. Fasting or limiting particularly fires up the NPY and drives the body to look for more sugars. So when the following eating opportunity happens, it can easily become a high-sugar gorge. For what reason is there such a compound drive for starches? How about we take a look at the basic job starches to play in the body—it will assist you with understanding the base yearning drive.

THE IMPORTANCE OF CARBOHYDRATES

Carbohydrates are the highest quality level of food energy available to the body. Cells work best when they get a specific unit of sugars, such as glucose, and even little deficiencies can cause issues. The mind, sensory system, and red blood cells depend solely on glucose for fuel. Due to the significance of glucose, the degrees of it in the blood are firmly managed by two hormones, insulin, and glucagon. There is an exceptionally restricted measure of sugar put away in the liver, as glycogen, that causes supply more glucose to the blood when levels get excessively low. However, this valuable fuel holds conventionally keeps going just three to six hours (except around evening time, when liver glycogen endures longer because the requirement for vitality is lower). How does this fuel hold get exchanged?

Eating starch-rich foods, that is. If the diet is deficient in sugars, the body needs to go to innovative energizing systems to supply indispensable vitality to the body. Protein predominantly from muscle will get dismantled and changed over to vitality, principally as glucose. It resembles taking wood from the system structure in your home to use as fuel in your chimney.

The wood will consume and give important fuel; however, it does as such at a significant expense. You start to lose the respectability of your structure! If you believe that eating a high-protein diet will keep this destroying from happening, it's not really. When you eat a deficient measure of vitality or starches, the protein from the eating regimen will likewise be redirected to be utilized as vitality. In this way, this "high-protein diet" is no protection. Instead, the protein is utilized as a costly wellspring of fuel, as opposed to for its expected use in the body. It resembles having a structure provider give loads of wood to modify your home.

If you are always utilizing that heap of wood to make campfires rather than to fix your home, you are still left with a frail structure. So also, protein is expected to keep up and construct muscles, hormones, compounds, and cells in the body. When starches and vitality are inadequate with regards to, protein is moved from its essential job to give fuel. A considerable lot of our customers accept that when we need more vitality, our bodies will, at last, start consuming fat. It doesn't work that way. Keep in mind, the cerebrum and different pieces of the body need starches solely for fuel.

Just a tiny part (5 percent) of the put-away fat can be changed over to a starch fuel. Then again, the body has a lot of compounds to change over protein to glucose. One reason individuals get more fit so rapidly on low-starch or fasting eats fewer carbs is that they are eating up their very own protein tissues as fuel. Since protein contains just half the same number of calories per pound as fat, it vanishes twice as quick. With each pound of body protein, three or four pounds of related water are lost. If your body were to keep on expending itself in light of current circumstances, demise would happen inside around ten days.

All things considered, the liver, heart muscle, and lung tissue—every fundamental cloth—are being singed as fuel. In any event, when the heart muscle is weakening, regardless, it needs to keep up a similar measure of work, with less power and at a more slow pulse. Generally, the tore apart heart muscle needs to work more enthusiastically with a littler, flawed motor; siphoning execution isn't diminished about the measure of heart tissue lost. In the long run, the body can change over put away fat to a type of usable vitality for the cerebrum and sensory system called ketones. This process is known as ketosis.

Ketosis is an adjustment to delayed fasting or starch hardship. Be that as it may, just about a portion of the synapses' can utilize these mixes for vitality. In this way, when fat is being utilized under these hardship conditions, the body's slender tissue (protein) keeps on being lost at a fast rate to supply glucose to sensory system cells that can't utilize ketones as fuel. The main concern? Sufficient sugars and vitality are significant! The Powerhouse Cell Theory Hunger signals are not influenced by low starches alone.

As indicated by crafted by cell analysts Nicolaidis and Even, the craving signal is produced by the general vitality need of the phone. When cell control is low, it will create a sign that actuates hunger. While cells get their vitality principally from starch, protein, and fat are calculated into the cell control condition, which could trigger yearning. For instance, regardless of whether one of your family unit apparatuses runs on unadulterated power, it could likewise get its vitality from batteries, or a gas controlled generator. They all give vitality, yet have various expenses and efficiencies. All supplements that give vitality (sugars, protein, and fat) in the long run get changed over to one widespread vitality division utilized by the cells, ATP. ATP is the synthetic vitality that powers the cells, and along these lines, our bodies. Nicolaidis and Even suggest that the appetite signal is activated by the general ATP need of the phone. To summarize—we need vitality. Vitality originates from food.

STEP BY STEP INSTRUCTIONS TO HONOR BIOLOGICAL HUNGER

It's too difficult to even think about hearing your appetite if you are never tuning in for it. The initial step regarding your natural appetite is to start to tune in for it. The ensemble of craving has numerous sounds that are shifted for various individuals. Similarly, as an ensemble director can recognize the voices of each instrument in an orchestra, you will, in the end, have the option to enter into explicit substantial sensations and what they mean. In the first place, you might have the option to perceive a clear greedy appetite; however, experience issues perceiving delicate food cravings.

Likewise, to the non-trained melodic ear, noisy cymbals may be anything but difficult to distinguish, yet it will require some serious energy and tuning in to get on the subtler voices of the bassoon or oboe. - Each time you eat, ask yourself: "Am I hungry? What's my craving level?" If the sentiment of yearning is difficult to distinguish, ask yourself: "When was the last time I at any point felt hungry? How did my stomach feel? How did my mouth feel?" Any mix of the accompanying can be experienced as yearning sensations or indications (running from delicate to insatiable):

- Mild murmuring in the stomach
- Growling within the stomach
- Light-headedness
- Difficulty concentrating
- Uncomfortable stomach torment
- Irritability
- Feeling faint
- Headache

The rhythmic movement of your appetite probably won't coordinate other people's—that is alright, its person. Take care not to get excessively hungry or greedy. If this is hard for you to check, a general rule is to go no longer than five waking hours without eating. This depends on the science of filling up your starch tank in the liver, which runs out each three to six hours.

We have seen that customers who go longer than five hours without eating will, in general, indulge at the following eating opportunity. To connect with the subtleties of yearning, it checks the beat of craving at ordinary interims. Check-in with your body, and basically ask, what's my appetite level? It's useful to do this each time you eat and between eating events. Keep in mind, despite the fact that this may appear hyperconscious; it's an engaged advance to get you reacquainted with your body and its science. We have utilized an assortment of apparatuses to enable our customers to check in with their appetite; however, one is especially useful and is somewhat less demanding.

Monitor your craving level each time you eat, prior, and then afterwards, utilizing the Hunger Discovery Scale. What example do you see developing? Is there a specific time during which you eat? Is there any connection between the amount you eat and the time allotment between eating? You may find that your eating style inclines toward snacking or brushing. Try not to be frightened.

If you eat modest quantities of food, for example, a tidbit or little meal, you may find that you are very hungry all the more frequently, for example, each three to four hours. In addition to the fact that this is ordinary, it might have favorable metabolic circumstances. Snacking considers (in which individuals are given various tidbits or smaller than usual suppers) have demonstrated that the arrival of insulin is lower in individuals bolstered snacking counts calories contrasted with bigger conventional meal s of indistinguishable calories. Insulin is a fat building hormone.

The more insulin released, the simpler it is for the body to accumulate fat. Once in a while, our customers get stressed when they all of a sudden vibe more hungry than expected—as though something isn't right. In any case, after looking into it further, they generally locate that two or three days earlier, they had a bizarrely light day of eating—not counting calories, however, just not a great deal of food. The body plays catch-up all alone terms. The vast majority of our customers experience issues recalling what they ate one day back, not to mention two days prior.

Research on kids has shown that they compensate for their wholesome needs in normal time from two or three days to seven days.

For what reason should grown-ups be any extraordinary? Actually, new research is starting to show the equivalent is valid for grown-ups. The body may do a portion of its vitality calibrating over a time of days, as opposed to from hour to hour. We discover this is particularly valid if, despite everything, you tend to eat diet kinds of food, for example, rice cakes or serving of mixed greens. You may feel full, yet the absence of vitality makes up for lost time with you. The body needs to redress.

Different Voices of "Craving" A typical mix-up with our more up to date customers is that they at first grasp the respect your yearning idea as an eating regimen mantra, "Thou will eat just when hungry." The issue here is that this unbending translation can leave you feeling as though you have disrupted a guideline, or fizzled If you eat for some other explanation than hunger. When you have a feeling that you have defied a norm, you can get maneuvered directly over into the diet mindset. Recognize that typical eaters don't generally eat just from unadulterated yearning, yet they keep up their weight.

- Taste Hunger. Now and then, individuals may eat basically because it sounds great or on the grounds that the event calls for it. We call this taste hunger. Ordinary eaters can acknowledge this—they don't see it as a major diet infringement. In about each culture, food assumes a significant job in rituals of entries and celebratory occasions. OK, chide a lady of the hour or lucky man for eating a bit of wedding cake when she or he was not very hungry? However, it's not uncommon for weight watchers to feel awful about any apparent food offense and afterwards feel like they should quit. Furthermore, that is when gorging regularly happens.
- Practical "Craving"— Planning Ahead. While it's critical to eat basically dependent on your organic

appetite, it's likewise imperative to be viable and not unbending. For example, suppose you are going to a play with companions that endures from 7:00 to 10:00 P.M. furthermore, your chance to eat is at 6:00 P.M. You may not be hungry at that point, yet you absolutely will be later. Do you stay there at the café and not eat, and let hunger move indirectly in the center of the play, just to come full circle in greedy yearning by the last demonstration? No. Eating a light meal or bite heretofore is a reasonable arrangement.

- Emotional Hunger. When you are really ready to recognize and accept your biological appetite, it gets simpler to explain why you need to eat. It isn't surprising for some of our customers to eat due to emotional yearning—to extinguish awkward feelings (for example, dejection, weariness, and outrage). Unexpectedly, a considerable lot of our customers are regularly flabbergasted that what they thought to be emotional eating was, in numerous cases, primal hunger eating. Be that as it may, the out-of-control feeling of overeating is almost indistinguishable, regardless of whether it was activated biologically or emotionally.

CHAPTER FIVE: FEEL YOUR FULLNESS

Tune in for the body signals that disclose to you are filled. Watch out for the signs that show you're comfortably full and can't eat anymore. Take a pause in the midst of eating and ask yourself how the food tastes, and what your present completion level is. The greater part of chronic dieters we have worked with has a place with the spotless-plate club. What's more, the vast majority of them state that they've done whatever it takes not to eat everything. It might appear that an obvious step to weight reduction is to regard your fullness, instead of to routinely "clean your plate."

However, leaving food can be hard to accomplish, particularly for chronic dieters. Dieting imparts a license to eat just at mealtime—when it is "legitimate." Ironically, this feeling of privilege strengthens a clean-your-plate attitude. This is especially valid for our customers who have tasted on over-the-counter fluid weight control plans, for example, Slim-Fast. (Fluid diet programs commonly have you drink a "refreshment supper" for breakfast and lunch, and afterwards "enable you to have a reasonable supper" of "genuine" food).

Naturally, the greater part of our patients for all intents and purposes licked their plates clean when allowed the chance to eat their one genuine meal. It isn't so much that they indulged; rather, they ate the entirety of their exact and "entitled" divides. Other diet plans utilizing normal food commonly offer little divides at meal s. This, as well, urges you to eat while you can. Who might leave any piece of food when amounts are pitiful? For instance, even frozen diet suppers float at around 300 calories (and regularly less), which ordinarily leaves you not exactly fulfilled. Truth be told, there is another pattern of frozen diet dishes offering considerably fewer calories—more like 200 calories for each bundle. This sort of eating scarcely cultivates connecting with your internal eating signals, particularly the signal of satiety. Rather, you eat everything.

Maybe you've hurled your diet plans out years prior, however now cautiously counting fat grams. You may discover, in any case, that you clean-your-plate with regards to eating without fat foods. We've had a few customers eat a whole bundle of without fat chocolate cake (or other sans fat treats) with cheerful surrender on account of the qualification factor. They would justify that "There's no fat so I can eat as much as I need." Unfortunately, without fat, it isn't really sans calorie. Be that as it may, the calories wouldn't be an issue if individuals were regarding their completion level. Obviously, different variables can easily condition you to finish each piece on your plate, including:

- Having been educated to complete everything on your plate by well-meaning parents.
- Respecting economics and the value of food—thou will not squander. Keep in mind, nonetheless, that whichever way the food can be squandered; on account of incessantly eating more than you need, it turns into an issue of increase in waist size.
- Having an instilled habit of eating to finish. Out of sheer habit, you finish a whole plate of food, or an entire burger, or an entire sack of chips, paying little heed to how very hungry or full you are. This is a dependence on outer prompts. You quit eating when the food is gone, paying little heed to the size of the underlying part.

- Beginning a meal (or snack) in an excessively covetous state. In this state, gobbling power is fired up, and it's very simple to sidestep typical satiety signals. Regardless of whether you don't clean your plate, it's still conceivable that you might be indulging, or bypassing your agreeable satiety level. With our customers who don't perfect their plates, we have frequently found that while there may, in any case, be food left on the plate, it took an awkward degree of totality to get them to quit eating. The issue is the failure to perceive comfortable satiety or to regard fullness.

THE KEY TO RESPECTING FULLNESS

Regarding fullness, or the capacity to quit eating since you have had enough to eat naturally, is based on giving yourself unqualified permission to eat. By what means can you or any dieter hope to leave food on your plate if you accept that you won't have the option to eat that specific food or meal once more? Except if you genuinely give yourself permission to eat again when you are hungry, or to approach that specific food, regarding totality essentially turns into a one-sided counting calories practice without roots. It won't grab hold.

The Intuitive Eater is based on preparing on how to quit eating when the individual in question has had only enough to fill the stomach, easily without being overfull. It's simpler to quit eating now and abandon food when you realize you can eat it again later.

RECOGNIZING COMFORTABLE SATIETY

We are amazed at how regularly our customers don't have the foggiest idea of what comfortable satiety level feels like. Goodness! However, they can, for the most part, portray incredible detail of how indulging or being overstuffed feels. However, information on what agreeable satiety feels like is frequently elusive, particularly to the chronic dieter. However, if you don't have the foggiest idea what agreeable satiety feels like, how might you expect to accomplish it? It resembles attempting to take shots at an objective while never observing it or knowing where it dwells. While regarding completion is the objective, it could easily be missed if you don't have the foggiest idea where to search for it, particularly when you have been adapted to clean your plate. Additionally, If you start eating when you are not hungry, it's difficult to tell when to stop out of totality. How would you envision agreeable satiety feels? Here are some regular portrayals offered by our customers:

- An unpretentious sentiment of stomach fullness
- Feeling fulfilled and content
- Nothingness—neither hungry nor full

The sensation is exceptionally personal and keeping in mind that we can depict it perpetually, it's similar to attempting to tell somebody what snow feels like. We can give you a smart idea or picture—however, it's something that should be experienced at the individual level, with the goal that you know how it feels, in your body.

HOW TO RESPECT YOUR FULLNESS

When you routinely clean your plate, your eating style effectively goes on autopilot—you eat until completion until the food is no more. To break this example of eating, we have thought that it was useful to be acutely mindful or hyperconscious of your eating. This implies being Conscious or aware of your eating experience. While you may positively know that you are occupied with the habit of eating, we find that somewhere close to the first bite and subsequent bites, there is a huge degree of knowing when you are full. Regularly the food isn't in any way, being tasted! In like manner, it's very simple to sidestep agreeable satiety. Here are a few models:

- I didn't know about how many treats I would eat at the motion pictures until all of a sudden, my hands were scratching at the sight of the unfilled box.
- I wouldn't consider parting a meal when eating out until my manager inquired as to whether I would part a course at her preferred eatery. Hesitantly, I concurred. Shockingly I was altogether happy with a large portion of a dish, realizing very well that had I requested the full segment, I would have eaten everything, out of sheer propensity.
- Once I open up a pack of any food, I intend to eat everything. God helping me, I'd leave a couple of goodies. I know I'm not in any event, tasting the food more often than not.

CONSCIOUS EATING

The underlying advance away from the visually impaired autopilot eating mode is Conscious eating. It's where you impartially watch your eating as though under a magnifying instrument. (Your Food Anthropologist voice will be useful here.) We have broken this phase into a progression of steps, which starts with taking a scaled-down break from eating. This will assist you with regrouping and evaluate where you are in your eating. It resembles the break that competitors and mentors take during a game to help improve their play or methodology. This is what to do.

Pause the meal or snack for a while. Remember that this break isn't a promise to quit eating. Or maybe, it's a promise to being under tight restraints with your body and taste buds. (If you felt that by stopping, you were committed to leaving food on your plate, you'd be hesitant to experience this progression. Truth be told, huge numbers of our customers who at first seemed uninterested in this progression later owned up that they were anxious about the possibility that they would need to prevent eating starting thereon.)

During this break, play out these checks:

TASTE CHECK:

We find that this check is normally pleasurable, which is the reason we like in any case, it. Ask yourself how the food tastes. Is it deserving of your taste buds? Or on the other hand, would you say you are proceeding to eat because the food is there?

SATIETY CHECK:

Ask yourself what your appetite or fullness level is. Is it accurate to say that you are as yet hungry, do you feel unsatisfied, or is your appetite leaving and would you say you are starting to feel fulfilled? To start with, this may appear to be an all in or all out process. Be tolerant, and recall, you are becoming acquainted with yourself from the back to front. Similarly, as you would not hope to become more acquainted with an individual more than one feast, how might you hope to comprehend your satiety level in one meal or bite? It will require some investment. Nonetheless, the more in the order you are with your yearning level, and the more you respect your appetite, the simpler this progression will be.

Make sure to be available to any answer. There can be extensive vacillation in your totality levels relying on the last time you ate and what you ate. If you find you're as yet hungry, at that point, continue eating. When you wrap up (whatever the sum), ask yourself where your totality level is currently. Did you arrive at agreeable satiety? Did you outperform it? By what amount? Utilize the Fullness Discovery scale to assist you with connecting. Note:

- Discovering your totality level will assist you in recognizing your Last-Bite Threshold. This is the endpoint. You realize that the chomp of food in your mouth is your last—finis! It might require some investment to get to this point. The more you have been detached from your body's feeling of totality, the more it will take to character this point. If you respect your appetite (Principle Two), it is a lot simpler to know totality. Assuming, be that as it may, you don't eat from organic hunger, how might you hope to prevent natural completion (or to try and recognize what it feels like)? It will be ideal if you show restraint toward yourself.
- Don't feel committed to leaving food on your plate. If you find that you have a degree of obstruction for this action, it might be from past

dieting experience. You might be feeling committed to leaving food on your plate, which is a remainder of the diet mindset. Keep in mind; there is no pledge to leave food on your plate. The dedication, rather, is to become more acquainted with your satiety level and your taste buds. It's impeccably typical, in any event, when you find your particular satiety level, to pick to indulge. That is alright. We have discovered that numerous customers keep on picking more food—they are as yet testing the "unequivocal authorization" to eat.

Sooner or later, when the originality wears off, you will find that it's very simple to leave food on your plate. It requires, be that as it may, a level of awareness—checking in with yourself. Be that as it may, if more often than not, you can perceive your completion, and regard it, it will have a significant effect in your capacity to keep up a characteristic weight.

INSTRUCTIONS TO INCREASE CONSCIOUSNESS

It's extremely hard to accomplish two Conscious things immediately. While you unquestionably may shuffle a zillion exercises, your brain centers basically around one. That is the reason, for instance, such huge numbers of individuals lock their keys in their vehicle. Their brains are centered elsewhere, for example, getting into the workplace on schedule, or emptying some food supplies. We find that to capitalize on(eating, it should be a Conscious action, at whatever point conceivable.

• Eat Without Distraction. Value and appreciate the eating experience whenever the situation allows. For instance, Adelle, a fast-paced, hard-determined legal counselor, constantly utilized her time, and would typically eat while accomplishing something different. Adelle would understand briefs while having lunch at work and would feast with a magazine at home. She stepped forward when she chose to have a go at eating without interruption when at home (she was excessively occupied at work to try and consider "simply eating" lunch). Adelle found that If she ate a meal or bite at home without participating in perusing, she would, for the most part, eat less.

Amazingly, she discovered that she ate less, not on the grounds that she was attempting to eat littler sums, but since she could identify her completion level a lot of sooner. She was excited that "easily" she was eating less food, feeling fulfilled without hardship, and not abstaining from excessive food intake. Adelle was happy to eat along these lines at home, yet didn't see it as reasonable for work—and this was advancement!

• Reinforce Your Conscious Decision to Stop. A considerable lot of our customers have discovered that when they choose to quit eating since they've arrived at the last-nibble edge, it's useful to plan something for make it a Conscious demonstration, for example, delicately pushing the plate forward a large portion of an inch or putting their utensils or napkin on their plate. This just helps them to remember their choice. Else, it might be very simple to guiltlessly snack on the rest of the food, despite the fact that you had no goal of doing as such. (If you experience difficulty with squandering food, take a stab at taking care of your scraps for tomorrow's lunch or meal or offering them to a vagrant.)

• Defend Yourself from Obligatory Eating. This typically implies working on saying, "No, thank you!" I never understood the criticalness of this demonstration until I (ET) went to an extremely exquisite mixed drink party in which there appeared to be one server for every visitor! The minute my hand was unfilled of food or drink, a very anxious server was there to offer more food or refreshment. I discovered it was such a great amount of simpler to state "yes," particularly If I was in a discussion. It took considerably more vitality to state "no." The equivalent is valid if you go to any capacity wherein there are benevolent "food pushers" from the thoughtful host to the offensive family member. A unique note of alert to those of you who appreciate wine by the jug at a decent café: A great server will frequently keep your glass full. Except if you are aware of that, you may drink more than you mean. Keep in mind; you are responsible for the amount to eat or drink.

THE FULLNESS FACTORS

"I just ate two hours prior—I regarded my craving and regarded my totality, so how might I be very hungry again unexpectedly early?" While the ebb and tide of satiety sign may appear to be bewildering, it's very ordinary to have various degrees of yearning and completion, particularly when you start tuning in to your body's eating prompts. There are, likewise, a few factors that influence totality. These components are both natural and educated. When you have a general comprehension of a portion of these satiety factors, it makes it simpler to confide in your body and feel your totality. The capacity to perceive agreeable satiety or completion can eventually decide how a lot of food will be expended in a supper. What's more, the measure of food eaten in a meal is impacted by these fullness factors:

• The measure of time that has taken a break you ate. The more regularly you eat, the less very hungry you will be. This has been seen as valid in snacking examines. These are pondering in which individuals f are given a few tidbits or little suppers for the duration of the day.

• The kind of food you eat. The macronutrients, protein, sugars, and fat impact is resulting in food admission by their commitment to the aggregate sum of food vitality in the stomach. Other food factors, for example, fiber, will likewise influence the fullness factor as a result of its mass and water retention properties. Protein specifically appears to have a suppressive/impact on consumption past its commitment to add up to calories, as indicated by a few investigations.

- The measure of food as yet staying in the stomach at the hour of eating. If your stomach is vacant, you will eat more than if some food is as yet present (from an earlier bite or feast).

- Initial yearning level. If you start a meal or nibble in a starving state, you are bound to gorge and abrogate satiety signals.

- Social impact. Eating with other individuals can impact the amount you eat. Studies have indicated that:

— The more individuals assembled at a feast, the more individuals will, in general, eat.
Eating with others increase the length of the meal.
— Eating more on weekends is ordinarily due to being around individuals.
— Dieters, be that as it may, have been appeared to eat less when they realize somebody is "watching" them. The equivalent is valid for non-dieters when they feast with a "model" eater. In one examination,

when the model eater ceased from eating, so too did the non-dieter.

There is a habit of disregarding or be diverted from biological signals in social settings. We have discovered that the way into the social issue is to keep making eating a Conscious action with deliberate food decisions. Obviously, there are numerous variables that impact how full you feel from eating. With such huge numbers of factors that apply impact on your eating, it ought to be nothing unexpected, at that point, that the measure of food you want to eat can and will change. A major key is to remain tuned in and to eat intentionally.

BE CAREFUL WITH AIR FOOD

Just pushing some food in your mouth like a pacifier to ease cravings for food may reverse the desired effect, and the comforting effect may not last long. This is particularly valid for "air food"— food that tops off the stomach yet offers little sustenance. Air food incorporates such low-calorie foods as air-popped popcorn, rice cakes, puffed rice oat, without fat saltines, „ celery sticks, and sans calorie refreshments. There's nothing intrinsically amiss with these foods. In any case, if you eat them hoping to get full, it will frequently take large amounts—and you may wind up waiting to pounce for something increasingly considerable to "top off the meal."

That's the place having a decent snack or meal, which incorporates a heavier sugar, some protein, or somewhat fat, is particularly useful, in case you're searching for a touch of "backbone," or the keep you going all day sort of feeling from eating. If then again, you realize you will go out for a breathtaking meal or to a gathering, and need only a touch of something to offer some relief from your craving; lighter foods may fill your need fine and moderately.

Foods with Staying Power Snacks or meals with a little fiber, complex starches, some protein, or even a little fat will help increment satiety. Amusingly, huge numbers of our ceaseless weight watchers avoid the very foods that could assist them with feeling increasingly fulfilled at suppers—complex starches. Here are some basic unacceptable food decisions and recommendations for how you can balance them to be all the more fulfilling. (There's nothing naturally amiss with these light foods, they just may not give backbone).

IMAGINE A SCENARIO IN WHICH YOU CAN'T STOP EATING.

If you find after time that regardless you are eating despite the fact that you are not very hungry, there's a decent possibility that you may be utilizing food as a method for dealing with stress. This isn't generally as clear and emotional as certain magazines recommend.

IMAGINE A SCENARIO IN WHICH YOU FEEL THERE'S SOMETHING MISSING.

If you've found what it feels like to feel easily full, but then feel that something is missing, it could be the fulfillment factor. This is so significant we've committed an entire rule to it—and talk about it in the next chapter.

CPSIA information can be obtained
at www.ICGtesting.com
Printed in the USA
LVHW082014220422
716976LV00004B/94

9 781803 035857